SIMPLE CHANGES:

THE BOOMER'S GUIDE TO A HEALTHIER, HAPPIER LIFE

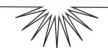

L. JOE PORTER, M.D.

Addicus Books, Inc.
Omaha, Nebraska

An Addicus Nonfiction Book

ISBN# 1-886039-35-6

Cover design by Jeff Reiner
Typography by Linda Dageforde
Author photo by Bob Murphy

This book is not intended to serve as a substitute for a physician, nor does the author intend to give medical advice contrary to that of an attending physician.

Library of Congress Cataloging-in-Publication Data
Porter, L. Joe, 1938-
    Simple Changes: the boomer's guide to a healthier, happier life / L. Joe Porter.
    p. cm.
    ISBN 1-886039-35-6 (alk. paper)
    1. Baby boom generation—Health and hygiene.   I. Title.
RA408.B33P67 1998
613'. 0434—dc21

                       98-33950
                       CIP

Addicus Books, Inc.
P.O. Box 45327
Omaha, Nebraska 68145
Web site: http://www.AddicusBooks.com
Printed in the United States of America
10 9 8 7 6 5 4 3 2 1

Contents

Acknowledgments

I wish to thank the following individuals for their assistance in the production of this book: Doug Porter, Dr. Gordon Gifford, Dr. Robert Thompson, Dr. Marc Miller, Polly Porter, Rev. Herb Hicks, Rev. Ray Vincent, Robert Glass, Marilyn Hooper, and especially Rhoda VanTassel.

Introduction

L ife is full of choices. Each morning you select what to wear and what to eat before leaving the house. You pick what route to take to work. Then what project to begin. You choose whether to smoke a cigarette, eat a candy bar, or enjoy an apple or banana on your break, and so on throughout the day.

Many of these choices, even the ones that are not good for you, are automatic because you have developed certain habits. The decisions are still there, but it is so much easier to go with what is familiar.

The good news is, you *can* change your habits. Practicing correct eating habits, exercise routines, and mental activities will soon bring you physical and emotional well-being. Once you grow accustomed to these healthy habits, you will continue to practice them as a lifestyle. Then you will hold the keys to a long and healthy life.

PART I
Weighing In, Eating Right, and Taking It All Off

1

Weigh Yourself Daily

Common Opinion: You can throw away your scales and track your weight-loss and fitness program by how well your clothes fit.

Medical Opinion: Your weight will vary a few pounds from day to day, and at different times during the same day. What you ate yesterday will not add extra pounds to your figure the following morning. However, what you eat will *eventually* show up there in real numbers.

Obesity kills. It also undermines your quality of life. Hypertension, diabetes, cancer, heart disease, gout, blindness, birth defects, trauma, gallbladder problems, bone and joint degeneration, and aches and pains are all attributed to obesity.

Charles Hennekens, chief of preventive medicine at Brigham and Woman's Hospital in Boston, points out that Americans are the fattest people on earth (except for the residents of a few Pacific islands). In fact, the United States is the heaviest society *in the history of the world.* The fattest age groups are men ages 50 to 69, and women ages 50 to 59. They are twice as likely to be obese as people in their 20s. Obesity among all males increased 72 percent from 1978 to 1995, with a 79 percent increase among males 50 to 69 years old. Among women the increase was 58 percent overall and 21 percent for those 50 to 69 years old.

Simple Change: You shouldn't overlook the use of a scale as a positive motivational tool in your health-and-fitness regime and as a daily reminder that you need to achieve an ideal weight.

P.S.: I was never extremely obese. Yet slowly, over the years, I gained forty pounds. That fact as well as a serious illness prompted me to develop a healthier lifestyle. I have changed several aspects of my daily routine, most notably one related to weight loss. Like so many of my patients, in the past I had tried multiple "diets." All were unsuccessful in keeping the weight off.

Why? By definition, a diet is bound to fail. A diet is something you stick with for a given length of time. It has a beginning and an end. The truth is, there is no end to achieving and maintaining your optimum weight.

I changed my eating habits stressing only one principle: "total calories in, total calories out." I lost forty pounds and five inches from my waist. This took approximately eight months. That was two years ago. I weigh myself every morning. I eat only when I'm hungry. I eat low-fat foods. Occasionally I do have a piece of pizza, but only one.

When my patients suggest that they are too old to change their habits, I simply relate my story and remind them that I am fifty-nine years old.

2

Be Hungry at Least Once Every Day

Common Opinion: You need to eat three balanced meals each day.

Medical Opinion: Your ideal weight is achieved and maintained by "total calories in, total calories out." There is nothing magical about eating at 7:00 A.M., noon, and 7:00 P.M. If you aren't hungry, don't eat. How many times do you go out to lunch with friends or colleagues just because you are asked? Do you reward yourselves with food for all your hard work every morning? Many people fall into an eating routine but are seldom hungry!

We often eat for the wrong reasons. We're bored. We're watching television. We're depressed. We're killing time. We need stimulation. Food is a pastime for many people.

If you are overweight, you need to burn more calories than you take into your body. Every day. Period. You can do this by eating sensible portions of low-fat, high-protein, high-fiber foods and by performing an adequate amount of activity.

Simple Change: Think before you eat. Make certain you are *really* hungry. If you aren't hungry, *don't eat!*

3

Look at Yourself Nude
in a Full-Length Mirror

Common Opinion: Looking at yourself in a mirror is to be avoided at all costs when you're trying to lose weight.

Medical Opinion: There's nothing like body image to spur you toward healthy eating habits. Recently, the editors of *The New England Journal of Medicine* stated that "the vast amount of money spent on diet clubs, special foods, and over-the-counter remedies, estimated to be on the order of $30 million to $50 million yearly, is wasted." Incentive, motivation, and feedback are strategies that weight loss centers use to divest you of your hard-earned money. Most centers also rely on medications as part of their total weight-loss plans.

Simple Change: Stand stark naked before a full-length mirror. Look at your entire body. With middle age comes the likelihood of increased fat around the middle. "Love handles," "spare tire," and "beer belly" are just a few of the unpleasant names we have assigned to this condition. If you don't like what you see, change it. Play mental games with yourself. Imagine your hips less full, a tummy that doesn't protrude, firmer upper arms, only one chin. Now keep that image with you as you go about your day. Try it. It works.

4

Start Your Day
with a Bowl of Bran Cereal

Common Opinion: Eating a high-fiber diet means starting every morning with a glass of bad-tasting liquid mixed from a powder.

Medical Opinion: Fiber comes in many forms and is essential to good health. A bowl of oatmeal contains 10 percent of your daily requirement of fiber. All-Bran has about 25 percent of your RDA. You can get fiber at every meal, of course. Grains, beans, crunchy vegetables, and citrus fruits are all good sources.

Fiber is extremely important in your diet. It can prevent cancer of the colon. Cancer of the colon is the second leading cause of cancer deaths among both men and women in the United States.

The Chinese diet contains three times more fiber than the typical American diet. As a result, the incidence of colon cancer in China is approximately two-thirds lower than in the United States. The Chinese also consume about 35 percent less protein, 50 percent less fat, and 30 percent fewer calories than do Americans. These factors may also reduce their risk of colon cancer.

Genetic factors also appear to influence the development of colon cancer. A study of 389 patients with colorectal cancer indicates that 15 to 20 percent had at least one relative who suffered malignancies of the large bowel. Fiber in the diet may be particularly important for those with a genetic predisposition to this type of cancer.

A number of studies have also shown that fiber-rich foods may help prevent breast cancer. One study demonstrates that a diet high in animal protein and fat and low in fiber coincides with a much higher risk of breast cancer, particularly among women under fifty.

Other studies at major medical centers suggest that a high-fiber diet may help prevent cancers of the esophagus, mouth, pharynx, stomach, endometrium (lining of the uterus), and ovary.

Here's the *really* big news: a high-fiber, low-fat diet may eliminate most hemorrhoids. It may well eliminate the need for laxatives among those suffering from chronic constipation.

Simple Change: Okay, if you absolutely can't eat bran cereal, then eat another high-fiber cereal every morning. Make certain that grains, fruits, and vegetables are well represented at every meal.

5

Eat Tuna Fish

Common Opinion: Eating meat is essential for good health.

Medical Opinion: Protein is essential in your diet, but it need not come from red meat. Tuna, salmon, mackerel, herring, anchovies, sardines, and lake trout are good sources of *omega-3 fatty acids*, or *EPA* (eicosapentaenoic acid). These substances are the best natural inflammation fighters. Inflammation is the source of pain in arthritic joints. Fish oils are also very helpful in producing the good type of cholesterol in your blood, reducing the amount of bad cholesterol.

Simple Change: Eat tuna or one of the other fish four times a week to get protein in your diet without the fat of red meat. Try making a tuna salad with chopped celery, chopped carrots, chopped onions, and no-fat mayonnaise. Eat this regularly with a green salad topped with no-fat dressing or with mixed fresh fruit. Drink a glass of skim milk and you have a .complete, ideal lunch. Occasionally substitute garlic/bean soup for the salad or fruit. Garlic has been shown to help lower cholesterol, fight infection, block cancer, and clear the arteries. This lunch is delicious, low in calories, low in fat, and high in protein and fiber.

6

Enjoy Baked Potatoes with No-Fat Gravy

Common Opinion: Potatoes are fattening. Gravies are even worse.

Medical Opinion: Potatoes are inherently good. They are excellent sources of fiber and nutrients. They contain no fat and a minimum of calories. But frying potatoes or drowning them in butter or sour cream changes the story drastically.

Simple Change: Eat baked potatoes often. When you eat them, eat the peel also. It's a good source of additional fiber and nutrients. Bonus: you can eat as many potatoes as you like.

P.S.: You can even add gravy! Several companies make no-fat gravy in three flavors: beef, chicken, and turkey. They're all good!

7

Include Fat-Free Yogurt in Your Diet

Common Opinion: Real men don't eat yogurt.

Medical Opinion: Yogurt contains little fat and is a great source of calcium and protein.

Simple Change: Try the many flavors of yogurt. Even if you think you won't like the taste, you will probably change your mind when you taste wonderful flavors like raspberry, peach melba, Key lime pie, and Boston cream pie.

P.S.: Some fat in your diet is essential to good health. It is needed to utilize fat-soluble vitamins. Limit your fat to 20 to 25 percent of your daily caloric intake (40 to 50 grams of fat on a 2,000-calorie diet) if you are at *ideal* *weight.* If you are overweight, reduce your fat intake to 20 to 30 grams of fat and adjust your total calories appropriately.

8

Use Mustard and Salsa on Your Food

Common Opinion: All condiments are created equal.

Medical Opinion: Mustard and salsa will increase your metabolism of the food they are eaten with by 20 percent. Therefore, you actually get 80 percent of the stated calories. Both mustard and salsa are low in calories and enhance the taste of foods. Low-fat foods like fish can be spiced up with sauces made of mustard or salsa.

Simple Change: Instead of putting mayonnaise on your next sandwich or dipping with high-calorie dips, substitute these two delicious toppings.

9

Drink Skim Milk

Common Opinion: You don't need to drink milk if you take a calcium tablet.

Medical Opinion: Most people are aware that milk is an excellent source of calcium. Most are not aware that milk contains other nutrients essential for healthy bones as you grow older. Drinking skim milk, rather than taking calcium tablets, is the best low-fat source of calcium, protein, vitamin D, and to a lesser extent, vitamin C.

Low bone density, or osteoporosis, may cause back pain, fractures of the vertebrae, wrist fractures, and hip fractures. Osteoporosis is a major health problem in the United States, affecting more than 25 million Americans and contributing to more than 1.5 million fractures each year. One of every two women over the age of fifty will suffer an osteoporotic fracture at some time in her life, as will one of every three men over the age of seventy-five. Even seemingly minor injuries may cause serious fractures with osteoporosis. As an orthopedic surgeon, I have found that osteoporotic fractures constitute a large percentage of my practice.

The National Heart, Lung, and Blood Institute recently studied carefully designed diets. A diet consisting of dairy products, two or three low-fat servings daily, combined with a diet rich in fruits and vegetables, lowered the blood pressure of hypertensive patients by an average of eleven points. This was on par with patients who instead took an antihypertensive medication.

Simple Change: Drink skim milk every day and exercise. For post-menopausal women, estrogen treatment or calcitonin may also increase bone density. Start early to prevent osteoporosis.

P.S.: Remember, when recipes call for milk, use *skim* milk. You don't need the extra fat that even 2 percent milk gives you.

10

Don't Salt Your Food

Common Opinion: Everything tastes better with salt. Besides, salt is important to your health.

Medical Opinion: Salt is an essential element in many of our metabolic processes. For most of us, salt intake is no problem. However, those who have a family history of *hypertension* (high blood pressure) and/or congestive heart failure should restrict the amount of sodium in their diets.

Many of us like the taste of salt but are unaware of just how much sodium many processed foods contain. For instance, one teaspoon of salt has about 600 milligrams of sodium—a quarter of your daily limit. One cup of rice has 840 milligrams of sodium, or 35 percent of your daily limit. Eight ounces of V-8 juice contain 620 milligrams of sodium, or 26 percent of your limit. Two tablespoons of Italian dressing contain 380 milligrams of sodium. Olive oil has *no* sodium.

Most people get plenty of sodium in their diet, without adding salt at the table.

Simple Change: Read the labels on processed foods before you buy them. Some of the high-sodium foods may surprise you. Your daily intake of sodium should be less than 2,500 milligrams.

If you must shake something on your food, use a salt substitute. Several on the market contain spices like dried parsley, basil, oregano, and cayenne. These spices will add zest to your meals.

11

Take a Multiple Vitamin Every Day

Common Opinion: For most people, taking vitamin supplements is a waste of time and money.

Medical Opinion: Vitamins contain antioxidants which enhance your body's natural defenses against *free radicals*—hyperactive atoms that can damage tissues and organs. These free radicals, that we take into our bodies from our increasingly polluted environment, may cause heart disease and cancer.

Many vitamin supplements contain *antioxidants*. The major antioxidants are vitamins A, C, and E. Other anti-oxidants found in some vitamin supplements include choline, ginseng, pumpkin-seed meal, oyster extract, L-cystine, garlic, selenium, glutathione, and bioflavonoids.

Each person requires different amounts of antioxidants at different ages, as well as for different activity and stress levels at the same age. The benefits of taking a daily vitamin supplement are myriad. Below are just a few.

Vitamins C and E in higher doses may help your immune system fight off colds and other viruses.

Vitamin E may also protect against Parkinson's disease and help slow Alzheimer's disease.

Vitamin A (beta-carotene) is important for healthy skin, hair, and mucous membranes. It also helps your night vision.

Vitamin B1 (thiamine) aids metabolism and promotes a healthy central nervous system and heart.

Vitamin B2 (riboflavin) promotes clear vision and is essential for growth.

Vitamin B3 (niacin) is important for your digestive system and stimulates blood circulation.

Vitamin B6 helps metabolize fat. It also facilitates the production of red blood cells and helps to balance the fluids in your body.

Vitamin B12 also helps in the production of red blood cells and promotes a healthy nervous system.

Folic acid facilitates the production of red blood cells and helps metabolize proteins.

Vitamin D is essential for healthy bones and teeth.

Vitamin K promotes proper blood clotting.

Simple Change: Read the labels of all vitamin supplements. Make certain they contain 100 percent of the U.S. RDA (Recommended Daily Allowance) of all the basic vitamins plus at least three times the RDA of vitamins C and E. They should also include substantial amounts of minerals like calcium, phosphorus, magnesium, and especially zinc. Take your vitamins as part of your daily routine.

12

Consider an Asprin a Day

Common Opinion: Aspirin is just a pain reliever.

Medical Opinion: Not simply a pain reliever, aspirin may save your life. Aspirin in low doses acts as a mild anticoagulant in your blood. The cheapest aspirin (acetylsalicylic acid) is just as effective as name brands. Interestingly though, high doses of aspirin are ineffective. Aspirin helps to prevent blood clots from forming in your arteries. Blood clots in your coronary arteries may cause heart attacks. Blood clots in the arteries that lead to your brain may cause strokes.

Patients who may have suffered a heart attack and who are immediately placed on aspirin have significantly fewer second heart attacks, strokes, and a lower death rate, according to the Second International Study of Infarction.

Aspirin is also one of the most effective anti-inflammatory and analgesic drugs. It is thought to inhibit the production of *prostaglandin*, an inflammatory substance in your body.

Simple Change: Ask your doctor about taking one aspirin tablet daily. Include aspirin on your list of medications. Remember to inform your physician, surgeon, or dentist that you are taking aspirin prior to any surgical or dental procedure.

P.S.: Use aspirin cautiously with children. Reye's syndrome, a rare but serious illness in children, may be caused by aspirin intake.

13

Reconsider Your Use of Alcohol

Common Opinion: Drinking a certain amount of alcohol may benefit your health without impairing your judgment.

Medical Opinion: True, according to recent reports, drinking a moderate amount of alcohol each day reduces your risk of cardiovascular disease. Yet even one drink alters your reaction time.

Alcohol abuse is a major factor in all types of accidental deaths, killings, family unhappiness, divorce, liver disease, osteoporosis, depression, and suicide. Most often, alcohol abuse results not from addiction but from habits that trigger drinking. For instance, you may stop into your favorite bar or club every afternoon after work. You do this to change your environment and/or

31

to meet your friends. As you walk in, your habit is to immediately order a drink. The environment triggers the response. Having a drink makes you feel comfortable. You have done it so many times before.

Reducing your intake of alcohol helps with weight loss. Twelve ounces of beer equals 160 calories. A gin and tonic equals 200 calories. Three ounces of sweet wine equals 150 calories. Three ounces of dry wine equals 100 calories. Alcohol use can also impair your judgment about eating nutritious, low-calorie foods.

Simple Change: How much is right for you? You be the judge. Once you decide, stick with it. That means if you have two glasses of wine every day, it *isn't* all right to have six drinks on Saturday, four on Sunday, and then go back to two drinks a day starting on Monday. If you do, you risk many other potential problems.

Recognize and change habits that trigger drinking. Please, *never* operate a motor vehicle after even a single drink.

P.S.:   I have quit drinking completely. I don't miss it at all. It is just one of the habits I changed to reduce weight.

There are many advantages to not drinking alcohol:
    1) easier weight loss and weight control
    2) no hangovers

3) a better relationship with your mate
4) extended evenings to pursue other interests
5) remembering what you ate for dinner
6) remembering who you talked to and what you said at a party
7) staying awake for an entire stage play or other event
8) better sleep patterns
9) more invitations to events where you can be the "designated driver"
10) more healthful decisions in your total lifestyle
11) eliminating "remorse and regret"
12) better-smelling breath
13) less chance of accidents occurring

PART II
Enhancing Your Physical Well-Being

14

Select a Clean-Air Environment

Common Opinion: Warnings about the air you breathe probably exaggerate the dangers. Besides, there's little you can do about bad air.

Medical Opinion: With the increasing industrialization of our cities, your lungs are constantly being bombarded with more foreign particles. Among the pollutants in air are carcinogens. Workers exposed to asbestos, benzene, coal-tar pitch, and uranium are more likely to develop lung cancer. Their risk of developing lung cancer is 60 percent higher if they also smoke cigarettes.

You may not live far enough away from a city or workplace to fully protect your pulmonary system. However, by making a conscientious effort, you can minimize the detrimental effects of urban air pollution.

37

Simple Change: Make surgical masks available in your home. Wear them when painting or when doing extensive housecleaning. The masks that surgeons wear in the operating room filter even the smallest particles. If you have any pulmonary problems, you will find these masks beneficial in cold weather or polluted air. These masks are readily available from most pharmacies or health-supply establishments.

If you both live and work in a city, try to spend as much time as possible indoors with air-conditioning. Drive an air-conditioned automobile. Don't smoke. Stay away from areas indoors where smoking is permitted. Practice aerobic exercises daily.

15

Wash Your Hands
Several Times Every Day

Common Opinion: Infectious diseases are passed primarily through the air.

Medical Opinion: Hand-to-mouth transmission is much more likely. Everything you come into contact with daily may expose you to disease-causing viruses and bacteria. Telephones, money, books, papers, pens, door handles, and playing cards, are all potential hazards. You may have seen pictures of Michael Jackson wearing a mask in public to guard against disease. He would have been better off to wear gloves on *both* hands.

Simple Change: Make it a habit to wash your hands frequently. Preferably, use an antibacterial soap. If you are in a public restroom, use the towel that you wiped your hands with to shut the water off and to open the rest room door. The last person to use the facilities may *not* have washed his or her hands.

It's a good idea for everyone to keep a box of disposable latex gloves around the house. Especially use them when handling raw meat. Uncooked meat contains bacteria that can be transferred onto your hands and then to other food you are preparing. If you don't use gloves, wash your hands with an antibacterial soap before handling other foods.

P.S.: We physicians wash our hands after seeing each patient in our offices. This not only protects us from disease-causing bacteria but also protects our patients from cross-contamination. More and more you will notice physicians and dentists using latex gloves in their offices.

16

Do Enough Exercise Three Times a Week to Get Mildly Short of Breath

Common Opinion: You need to exercise every day to get the kind of workout you need to stay healthy.

Medical Opinion: You don't need to spend your hard-earned cash to exercise your heart and lungs. Any activity that produces mild shortness of breath is just as effective as using a stationary bike or treadmill. As you get older, however, non-loading exercises like swimming or bicycling will give you the advantage of cardiovascular training without wear and tear on your joints. I won't suggest a target heart rate for you while exercising, nor a specific time frame. Just get short of breath, then continue the activity a few minutes.

The advantages to following a regular exercise regimen are legion.

- Exercise has been shown to increase the good type of cholesterol in the blood and to decrease the harmful type, thus reducing your chances of developing arteriosclerosis, which can lead to heart and blood-vessel disease. Your risk of high blood pressure and diabetes are also greatly diminished by regular exercise.

- Exercise promotes strong, well-toned muscles that will protect your joints from wear and tear as you undertake your daily activities. Firm muscles will also protect your joints from injuries that can occur from strenuous exercise, sprains, and strains.

- Exercise may improve your emotional health. Learn to vent your aggressions from a stressful day in short bursts of physical activity.

- Exercise promotes relaxation and enhances sleep.

- Exercise improves sexual function by reducing stress.

- Exercise strengthens the bones, increasing their density.

Simple Change: Do a little extra exertion every day. Walk up a flight of steps, or down three or four, instead of taking an elevator. Park your car a block away from your usual parking spot and walk. Try walking to at least some of the golf holes instead of riding in the golf cart the whole way.

To get in the habit of exercising, first write it down in your weekly planner. Make an appointment with yourself. This is one appointment you must never break or you'll feel guilty.

Right now, you may follow your workday with a couple of drinks or watching TV, then dinner, and finally more "down time" in your favorite chair. Instead, try eating your last meal earlier (at 5:30 or 6:00 P.M.), followed by some form of physical exertion, then a rest period, and then go to bed. Exercising after your evening meal will promote more restful sleep.

P.S.: I have found that my golf score has improved by simply walking from one shot to the next. This exercise allows me to evaluate the position of the ball, the difficulty of the lie, and the distance I want to hit the next shot. No longer do I ride up to the ball from some circuitous route on a golf cart. Okay, I admit that state-of-the-art advancements in golf equipment help a little. The biggest Big Bertha driver has a head so big that it's impossible to hit anything but a good drive.

43

17

Avoid Back Pain

Common Opinion: Frequent backaches are just a sign of aging. Nothing can be done about them.

Medical Opinion: Standing strains your back. You can walk for a far longer time than you can stand still. During prolonged standing, the muscles that hold your spine erect become tired and allow your lower back and hip to sag forward, causing a backache.

There are several simple rules to follow to prevent back pain. There is a right way and a wrong way to do everything, even sitting and standing. Even if your back is healthy and strong, you will minimize your chances of developing an injury or strain if you perform daily activities properly.

Simple Change: Stand with your hips flexed to remove the strain on your back. You can accomplish this by simply placing one foot on a stool or a step. That is why a rail is usually found under the bar in a tavern.

When sitting, avoid sway in your lower back. If you are sitting at a desk or table, sit in a relaxed position, but not in a slouch. Your weight should be evenly distributed. You should not be twisted in the chair. Your back should be supported by the back of the chair. Your feet should be firmly on the floor. Your chair should be firm, not soft. If it is too high, your hips will be higher than your knees. This will only cause your back to sag forward, increasing the strain.

When driving your car, do not sit with the seat too far back. If your legs are straight, your lower back will curve forward. Instead, adjust your seat so that your knees are raised and your back is straight.

When lifting objects, never lean forward without bending your knees. As you rise, straighten without arching your back. Most of the effort will come from your legs. The same rule applies if you are carrying an object. Never lift anything above the level of your elbows. This will only throw your balance off and force you to arch your back to keep the weight of the object from pulling you forward.

18

Engage in at Least Two Hours of Activity after Your Evening Meal

Common Opinion: There is nothing wrong with "vegging out" in front of the TV all evening as a reward for working hard all day.

Medical Opinion: You will find that physical and mental activities in the evening hours will promote more restful sleep. Good sleeping habits are essential for good physical and mental health.

Simple Change: Continue activities after your evening meal so that you continue burning calories. Remember, weight control depends on only one thing: "total calories in, total calories out." Also, if you have a busy schedule, this may be your only chance to undertake the light exercise program that I have suggested.

Get into the habit of *not* turning on the TV. Get your evening news from the daily newspaper. Find entertainment in physical and mental exercises.

19

Understand Arthritis

Common Opinion: Arthritis only afflicts the elderly. Not much can be done to prevent arthritis or to relieve its effects.

Medical Opinion: As you age, your joints tend to get a little stiffer. This limits your range of motion. In turn, limited motion limits the nutrition to the edges of the cartilage in your joints. If your nutrition is poor, the edges of the cartilage begin to degenerate. This result is *arthritis* (also called *osteoarthritis* or *degenerative arthritis.*) Fifty million Americans have this problem.

So force those joints and milk that cartilage. Your cartilage and thus your joints will stay healthier.

Arthritis is very different for different individuals. The same amount of cartilage damage in one person may cause a great deal of agony but in the next person may cause little or no pain, swelling, or tenderness. Also, a patient may exhibit different degrees of arthritic symptoms on different days. People also respond differently to various medications and other arthritic treatments.

If you suffer from arthritis, visit your physician. Find out what type of arthritis you have. Some types of arthritis, like *gouty arthritis*, can be completely controlled with medication. Other forms, like *rheumatoid arthritis*, may require aggressive treatment in the form of prescription drugs, specific exercises, or in some cases, surgery.

Simple Change: Take all your joints through a full range of motion every day. Range-of-motion and stretching exercises are most beneficial for preventing and treating arthritis. Strenuous exercise, however, may precipitate or worsen arthritis.

Be careful about buying fad to prevent or treat arthritis. The fad diets include eliminating fruits, herbs, dairy products, and preservatives. Some diets suggest eating alfalfa in high doses or eliminating vegetables in the nightshade family such as eggplant, bell peppers, potatoes, and tomatoes. Fad equipment includes gold bracelets, magnets, and other "arthritic jewelry." Symptoms of osteoarthritis go through peaks and valleys naturally over time. If you find yourself in an arthritic "valley," bury a dish rag from your grandmother's kitchen in the backyard, and if your symptoms improve, you just may believe that you have discovered a cure for arthritis.

20

Cover Up When You're Out in the Sun

Common Opinion: Tanning is okay if it is done sparingly.

Medical Opinion: There is no such thing as a safe tan. True, a tan provides some protection against ultra-violet rays. Yet the dangers using a suntan far outweigh the minimal protection a tan offers.

Whenever your skin is exposed to the sun, some damage occurs. This is a cumulative effect. Eighty percent of skin damage by the sun usually occurs before age twenty. It is worthwhile to assume the sun is like a giant nuclear reactor. Now, ask yourself how much time you should spend basking in the glow of a nearby nuclear plant. None. The same is true of the sun. There is no safe exposure. People with red hair, green eyes, and/or fair skin are at the greatest risk.

The sun's ultraviolet rays cause skin cancer. About 1.2 million Americans get skin cancer each year. Ultraviolet rays are most intense between ten in the morning and three in the afternoon. The ozone layer protects against ultraviolet rays. However, the ozone layer decreases in the fall and winter, offering less protection.

Look for early warning signs of skin cancer: a sore that doesn't heal, any changes in the size or color of a wart or mole, or the development of any unusual pigmented area. Early detection and prompt treatment virtually assure a complete cure for the two most common types of skin cancer, *basal cell carcinoma* and *squamous cell carcinoma*. The more serious *melanoma* has a five-year survival rate of 85 percent.

So-called age spots, wrinkles, dry skin, and small growths are often attributed to aging. But if you were to check the skin on a person's buttocks, you would usually find no changes in that area. Therefore, such changes are typically the result of long-term exposure to the sun.

Applying protective creams and lotions is crucial. Factor 15 sunscreens are usually considered adequate. However, stronger creams and lotions, up to factor 60, are available.

Simple Change: Remember this good advice: "slip, slap, slop." Before you go out into the sun, first "slip" into protective clothing. "Slap" on a hat. "Slop" on sunscreen. The tighter the weave of fabric, the more protective clothing is. Wet clothes lose 30 percent of their protective factor. Wear a hat with a wide brim to protect the nose, ears, and lips. Sunglasses are extremely important since your eyes, too, may be damaged by the sun. Some cataracts and degeneration of the lining of the eye may occur.

P.S.:   The skin is the largest organ of your body. When spread out, it covers twenty square feet. Protect it!

21

Buckle Your Seat Belt

Common Opinion: Seat belts aren't necessary when you are running short errands. Besides, buckling up is not really necessary if you have air bags.

Medical Opinion: Every year, hundreds of families and friends mourn the loss of loved ones who die in motor vehicle crashes. Many states require all front seat occupants to wear their seat belts, but the laws are never adequately enforced.

Studies show that wearing a seat belt may increase a person's chance of surviving a motor vehicle crash by 50 percent. And most car accidents occur within twenty-five miles of home.

Don't let air bags give you a false sense of security. Researchers at the University of Medicine and Dentistry of New Jersey checked the medical records of crash victims involved in motor vehicle accidents. All were in cars equipped with air bags. Of the 38 crash victims in the study, 16 weren't wearing seat belts. Six of the unbuckled patients died. Only 1 of the buckled patients died. Of the 31 survivors, those who weren't wearing seat belts spent twice as long in the hospital and had suffered far worse injuries.

In an airplane, unexpected turbulence may throw you around or even out of your seat, causing severe injuries.

Simple Change: Refuse to start your car until you and all passengers are buckled up. Also, remember to keep your seat belt fastened on airplanes at all times.

P.S.: I value freedom and independence. However, the benefits of wearing a seat belt far outweigh any perceived intrusion on individual rights. Those who do not wear their seat belts only burden the rest of us with more workers' compensation claims, bigger insurance premiums, and ultimately higher health care costs.

Sandra Rosenbloom of the Drachman Institute at the University of Arizona offers excellent suggestions for safe driving.

- Pay attention. The average driver must make about twenty major decisions for every mile driven.

- Make sure you can see the road ahead clearly. A sixty-year-old needs ten times as much light as a twenty-year-old to see properly. Keep your eyes moving. Glance into your rearview mirror often, scanning both the roadway and the areas beside it. Use both your inside and outside rearview mirrors. Keep your windshield clean.
- If you're short, consider using seat cushions. You should sit high enough so that your shoulder is in line with the top of the steering wheel. Make sure the headrest is adjusted for your height, for it could prevent serious neck injuries in a crash.
- Plan your driving. Avoid driving at the busiest times of the day on heavily congested roads.
- Keep a three-second safety margin between your car and the one in front.
- On unfamiliar trips, take a "navigator" with you to refer to maps and to help you watch for road signs. Avoid distracting chitchat.

22

Don't Ignore Changes in Yourself: Signs of Stroke, Diabetes, and Injury

Common Opinion: Mild aches and pains simply mean you are growing older.

Medical Opinion: You must be alert to subtle signs that persist because they may be symptoms of serious physical problems.

A recent survey in the *Journal of the American Medical Association* finds that 43 percent of 1,880 adults surveyed cannot identify even one of the five warning signs of an impending stroke. Stroke is the third-leading cause of death in the United States, following heart disease and cancer. Six hundred thousand people a year suffer a new or recurrent stroke. About 160,000 people die from strokes each year. Knowing the early signs of a stroke is extremely important because there is a drug that will reduce damage if given within three hours of the onset of symptoms. This drug is *TPA*, which actually breaks up blood clots that cause a stroke. With TPA treatment, more than a third of patients may enjoy near-complete recovery.

Some risk factors can't be changed. These include increasing age, race, diabetes, previous stroke, and family medical history. However, you can treat several conditions to reduce your risk of a stroke.

- high blood pressure
- heart disease
- cigarette smoking
- heavy intake of alcohol
- mini-strokes, or *transient ischemic attacks*. (*TIAs* last less than five minutes and are very important warning signs.)

Simple Change: Learn the five warning signs of stroke.

- sudden weakness or numbness of the face, arm, or leg, especially on one side
- sudden dimness, decreased vision, or loss of vision, particularly in one eye

- sudden difficulty speaking or understanding speech
- unexplained dizziness, unsteadiness, loss of balance, or falls
- sudden severe, unexplained headaches

Learn the warning signs of diabetes.

- frequent urination. (Patients frequently pass large amounts of urine, typically in excess of three or four liters every twenty-four hours. Among children previously toilet trained, bed-wetting may be the first sign of the juvenile form of this disease.)
- inordinate thirst
- increase in appetite
- unexplained weight loss
- loss of strength
- drowsiness after eating which may be abnormal among older people with diabetes
- failing vision

Also, don't ignore a minor injury. Even a simple sprain of your knee or ankle, if not allowed to heal properly and completely, may eventually become a chronic problem. It could even lead to post-traumatic arthritis.

P.S.: As a team physician, I cannot emphasize enough to coaches and athletic trainers the importance of taking injuries seriously. Following an injury to a key player, the first thing a coach often wants to know is exactly how many days the player will be out of practice. With my own teams, coaches and trainers have learned that there is no set number of days a player will be sidelined. It is the *extent* of the injury, not the type of injury, that counts. Be patient. It may take several visits before a physician can predict the severity of a player's injury. If the severity of the injury is ignored and a player returns too early, a chronic injury may develop.

23

Take Medicine Only As Prescribed

Common Opinion: If one pill makes you feel better, then two pills should make you feel twice as good!

Medical Opinion: Care should be used when taking all pills, especially narcotics. Some non-narcotics like Darvon and Talwin, if not addictive, may still make you dependent on larger doses or more frequent use for the desired effect. Chronic back or neck disorders frequently lead patients to get hooked on analgesics. You can also grow dependent on muscle relaxants. For back and neck disorders, ask your doctor about *nonsteroidal anti-inflammatory drugs* (*NSAIDs*). These drugs help you overcome the inflammation causing the pain.

Very few drugs have to be taken as a matter of life and death. The dosages of many medications may be safely decreased until you consult your physician. In fact, most can be safely discontinued until at least the next day. If you have questions about possible side effects, contact your physician immediately.

It certainly goes without saying that "recreational use" of any drug will eventually result in poor health and an early death. Drug dependency and addiction are among the most serious problems in the United States today.

Simple Change: Before you leave your doctor's office, make sure you know the *name* of the prescribed medicine, *why* you are taking it, what *results* you can expect, *how often* you should take it, and *all* possible side effects, including the potential of addiction. Also you should understand exactly *when* to take the prescription.

When you visit the pharmacy, ask your pharmacist to answer these same questions and to give you a written statement of everything he or she has told you. Follow these instructions to the letter.

When taking antibiotics, finish the entire prescription in order to completely rid your body of the bacteria. Do not stop just because you are feeling better. If you stop too soon, the infection may return.

24

Carry a List of Your Medications, Allergies, and Illnesses

Common Opinion: In an emergency, either you or your family will always be able to relate your medical history to the medical personnel taking care of you.

Medical Opinion: Although older persons make up 13 percent of the U.S. population, they use 36 percent of all prescription drugs. Therefore, it is imperative to be very aware of medicines, dosages, and drug interactions as you grow older. J. F. Moellar and N. A. Mathiowetz report in a recent *Health and Human Sciences Journal* that 87 percent of older patients are taking at least one prescription medication and three over-the-counter drugs each day.

There is a direct relationship between the number of drugs taken and a higher risk of adverse drug interactions. Approximately 19 percent of hospital admissions of older persons are attributable to drug interactions. Each year, drug interactions account for a significant number of falls that require operations to repair fractures.

Hospitalized patients and those in nursing homes are typically taking six to nine drugs, according to the 1998 edition of *Practical Ambulatory Geriatrics*. Adverse reactions to certain drugs may be due to the increased sensitivity of older persons or to possible interactions of certain frequently prescribed drugs. One example is the adverse reaction that occurs if the blood thinner Coumadin is taken with aspirin.

Simple Change: Prepare a list of your medications, allergies, and illnesses now. Assemble this list with the aid of your doctor and pharmacist. Carry it with you at all times. If you have a life-threatening disease such as diabetes, it is also a good idea to wear a medical ID bracelet imprinted with the name of the disease and your medication. When listing your medications, also state the dose and the dosage schedule. Be sure to update your list when you change medications or change doses.

Also include the name, address, and telephone number of your family physician and your choice of a general surgeon, should you need one. Write down your choice of hospital or medical center, if time allows, should an accident occur. Include the name, address, and telephone number of whom to contact in case of an emergency.

25

Get Your Z-Z-Zs

Common Opinion: If you have trouble sleeping, making it through the day on caffeine and adrenaline is a fact of life. There's not much you can do about it.

Medical Opinion: Sleep is extremely important for many reasons. Obviously, you need adequate amounts of sleep for physical well-being. The number of hours of sleep required varies from individual to individual. Also, you may find that some nights you need more sleep than other nights, depending on your activity during the day. There is no simple test to assess how much sleep a person requires. Instead, optimal wakefulness is the best indicator. "Enough" sleep enables a person to function competently during the day without much drowsiness during prolonged, monotonous, quiet situations.

More than 100 million Americans, according to the American Sleep Disorders Association, regularly fail to get a good night's sleep. Some eighty-four sleeping disorders result in diminished quality of life and personal health.

For most people, caffeine alters sleep patterns. It may keep you from going to sleep or wake you prematurely. It also is a strong diuretic, so you may have to interrupt your nice sleep pattern with a trip to the bathroom in the middle of the night.

Evidence suggests that heart disease and gastric acid production are linked to heavy caffeine users. Don't forget that other drinks and foods besides coffee and tea also have caffeine. Most soft drinks and chocolate contain caffeine.

It has been shown that the body releases the greatest amounts of human growth hormone while you are asleep. This hormone helps your cells divide and grow, especially in childhood. It also helps all your organs repair damaged tissues. Sleep deprivation over long periods of time may disrupt any of your vital functions.

Your immune system is not nearly as efficient if you are deprived of sleep for long periods of time. This may set you up for all sorts of physical problems, from minor infections to cancer.

Lower back pain, a common malady, has many interrelated causes. Bad sleeping habits are among the most common. An uncomfortable or worn-out mattress may result in fitful sleep. Simply sleeping on a firm mattress in the correct position may relieve your aching back, and allow you to get that much-needed good night's sleep.

Simple Change: Below are more tips for a good night's sleep.

- Sleep only as much as you need to feel refreshed the next day.
- Get up at the same time every day.
- Exercise daily.
- Insulate your room against sound and light.
- Keep the temperature of your bedroom comfortable.
- Avoid hunger or excessive fullness at bedtime.
- Avoid excessive liquids in the evening to minimize your nightly trips to the bathroom.
- Avoid caffeinated beverages in the evening.
- Avoid the chronic use of tobacco.
- Avoid alcohol, especially in the evening. Although alcohol may help you fall asleep more easily, it will later fragment your sleep.
- If you feel angry and frustrated because you cannot sleep, get out of bed, go to a different room,

and do something different. Do not try harder and harder to fall asleep.

- If you find yourself looking at the clock at night, turn it so that you cannot see it.
- Turn your mattress every three to four weeks. One time turn it over, the next time turn it end to end.
- Break yourself of the habit of sleeping on your stomach. Sleep on your back with a small pillow under your head (or none at all). Otherwise, sleep on either side with your knees and hips slightly flexed and a moderate-sized pillow under your head. These two positions will allow your spine to assume its ideal posture.

26

Don't Smoke Cigarettes

Common Opinion: Smoking may be bad for your health, but maybe you can beat the odds.

Medical Opinion: Like obesity, cigarette smoking is a known cause of disease. The more cigarettes you smoke, the more likely you are to develop lung cancer, emphysema, and/or heart disease. Very few people are able to smoke occasionally.

Simple Change: Don't start smoking cigarettes. If you smoke now, stop. There are many methods and medications on the market to help you quit. Choose them carefully. Nicotine gum, nicotine patches, and nicotine nasal sprays may protect your lungs from abrasive tar and nicotine but will not protect your other organs.

The American Lung Association, the American Cancer Society, and the American Heart Association offer good advice on how to stop smoking.

Understand that nicotine is an addictive stimulant that makes people feel better. If you want to stop smoking, you first have to overcome the addiction. It takes more than just a simple change of habit. You have to *want* to quit with all your heart and soul. Many of us have quit because of an associated disease, a heart arrhythmia in my case. This may make your decision easier. In any event, you will need preparation, motivation, and perseverance to reach your goal.

Assess *why* you smoke. Stress? Drinking alcohol? Peer pressure? The better you understand yourself, the more successful you will likely be at quitting.

Choose a strategy that best suits you. Your approach might emphasize behavioral changes (chewing gum or exercising), nicotine replacement (nicotine gum, nasal spray, or patches), medications, or alternative treatments (hypnosis or acupuncture).

Set a date to quit.

If you relapse into smoking, don't give up. Many people do this. Just set another date and stop again. Practice makes perfect.

P.S.: There are many other reasons for not smoking. You save money. You have fewer holes in your clothing, rugs, and furniture. You reduce your risk of burning to death in bed. It is more likely that your mate will want to kiss you or even get very close to you. Your clothing will smell better. So will your hair. You will get better seating in restaurants. You won't have to go outside in the cold at intervals. Your car will smell better. Your teeth will look better.

27

Get a Flu Shot Every Year

Common Opinion: Unless you are elderly or chronically ill, getting a flu shot is a bad idea. You can actually get the flu from the shot.

Medical Opinion: In recent years there is no evidence of a live influenza virus being given. What about your neighbor who got the flu from getting a shot? It didn't happen. He or she was either exposed to the flu before the shot or had an allergic reaction to the vaccine.

Many deaths each year occur not only from influenza and pneumonia but also from cardiopulmonary and other chronic diseases exacerbated by the flu. It is estimated that greater than 20,000 influenza-related deaths occurred during each of nine different flu epidemics in the United States from 1972 to 1992. Greater than 40,000 influenza-related deaths occurred during just four of those epidemics.

Each year's influenza vaccine contains the three virus strains (usually two type A and one type B) that are likely to circulate in the United States in the upcoming winter.

Simple Change: Sure, you've heard on TV that flu shots are recommended for the elderly, chronically ill, and health care providers. So why not you, too? It's cheap, even free, at many county and city health clinics. It's almost painless. It may prevent a week of illness, more if you were to develop complications like pneumonia. The optimal time for vaccination is usually October through mid-November. If the shot is given too early, the antibody levels may begin to decline by the peak of the flu season, rendering the vaccine less effective.

28

Men Over 40: Get a Yearly PSA Test for Prostate Cancer
Women Over 40: Get a Yearly Pap Smear and Mammogram

Common Opinion: Prostate cancer in men and uterine cancer in women are the diseases of old people.

Medical Opinion: One of every two women will develop cancer in her lifetime. Breast cancer is the most commonly diagnosed cancer among women. It kills 44,000 a year. For men, the chance of developing cancer is one in three. Men have a one-in-six chance of developing prostate cancer.

Early detection of cancer results in a high rate of cure. Evidence suggests that some cancer cells may be present in certain organs very early in life or even at birth. These cells may remain dormant until they are triggered later on in life by some stimulus and begin to multiply rapidly. Frequent examinations and testing are a must if cancer is to be detected early and treated successfully.

Precancerous signs and conditions must be taken seriously. Seek medical advice immediately. For example, rectal bleeding or changes in bowel habits should direct you to a physician for examination. If polyps are the cause of the bleeding, frequent reexaminations, as suggested by your doctor, should be performed.

Other early warning signals of cancer are a sore that doesn't heal, any unusual bleeding or discharge, a thickening or lump in the breast or elsewhere, indigestion, difficulty swallowing, obvious changes in a wart or mole, a nagging cough, and hoarseness.

If you suspect cancer, your health care provider will order a thorough investigation after he or she performs a routine physical examination. He may conduct a *proctosignmoidoscopy* (exam of the rectum and large bowel with a scope), *mammography* (x-ray of the breasts), or a *Pap test* (microscopic examination of cells from the cervix).

Simple Change: If you have any of these warning signs of cancer, see a physician or health care provider without delay. If it turns out not to be cancer, you will have peace of mind. This reassurance can alleviate anxiety from your life and add to your general well-being.

If cancer is present, your chances for a cure will increase by receiving prompt treatment. Your physician may then order a *biopsy,* in which a sample of tissue is removed and examined microscopically. You may also be referred to a cancer specialist, an *oncologist.*

29

Go to Church

Common Opinion: There is no relationship between good health and going to church or developing our spiritual self.

Medical Opinion: There is much we physicians do not know about spiritual healing. We *do* know for sure that part of the healing power we possess resides in the confidence that our patients have in us. There is a growing awareness of the interrelationships among thought, emotion, hormones, T cells (cells that fight infection), and the immune system. Scientists are recognizing the inseparable oneness and organic connectedness of life.

Cognitions beliefs, desires, and dreams give rise to emotional and physiological states. Medical researcher and psychiatrist David Larson reports in the *American Journal of Psychiatry* that more than 90 percent of the psychiatric literature he reviewed over twelve years shows a link between religion and good mental health. Religion proved to be protection against suicide, drug and alcohol abuse, and depression. Purdue University sociologist Kenneth F. Ferraro discovered that active participants in religious activities report significantly higher states of health and well-being than those who don't.

Psychologist Arthur Stone of the Medical School of the State University of New York at Stony Brook argues that uplifting events such as worship and fellowship have a stronger positive impact on the immune function than upsetting events do a negative one. In a study of 1,700 older Americans, researchers at Duke University Medical Center found that those attending religious services had stronger immune responses. About 60 percent of the men and women surveyed attended religious services at least once a week. Blood tests show that regular attendees were less likely to have high levels of an immune-system protein linked to age-related diseases. This study suggests attending a church has a direct positive effect on the immune system.

Dr. Dale Matthews, a professor at Georgetown Medical School, has studied the effects of prayers on recovery from heart problems. Half of the nearly 400 patients in his study were subjects of prayers, while the other half received no prayers. The patients who received prayers suffered half as many complications as those who didn't. Dartmouth Medical School tracked how patients' own prayers helped them recover from bypass surgery. The overall death rate six months after surgery was 9 percent. For churchgoers it was 5 percent. For those ranked as deeply religious, none died.

Simple Change: If you are a believer in a Supreme Being, then you know why. If you are an agnostic, go to church, learn, then go home and think about what you've heard. If you are an atheist, go and sing loudly, for it will increase your lung capacity.

P.S.: As a surgeon, I know that a visit by a patient's pastor or priest the night before surgery is more effective than any medication I can prescribe.

PART III
Enhancing Your Emotional Well-Being

30

Kiss Your Parents and Children Every Time You See Them

Common Opinion: Showing emotion to your parents and children is often embarrassing and awkward.

Medical Opinion: Remember, you don't have very long to show affection to the people you love. Your parents will pass on all too soon. Your children will all too soon not let you kiss them.

Simple Change: Don't be afraid to express affection to those you love. Kiss them often. And yes, men, kiss your father and sons. Even if they don't want to, do it anyway. And tell them you love them.

P.S.:   Fond memories of your positive relationships with your parents will help you overcome stressful situations as you face the problems of parenthood. Many psychologists believe we are the children within ourselves. That is, we tend to treat ourselves and our emotions, both positive and negative, as our parents would have treated us. "The child is father of the man," writes the English poet, William Wordsworth.

Age differences among your loved ones will seem less and less as the years go by. Therefore, establishing close relationships with your children will form the basis for long, rewarding friendships.

31

Spend Fifteen Minutes at Midday in a Quiet Room with Your Eyes Closed

Common Opinion: Successful people are always on the go, sometimes at a frenetic pace. That's life.

Medical Opinion: Quiet reflection can lower your stress. Lowering your stress means your immune-response systems can function more efficiently, decreasing your risk of illness. Also, recent evidence suggests that eliminating or reducing the stress associated with cancer may actually result in a higher rate of cure.

Simple Change: Spend fifteen minutes at midday in a quiet room with your eyes closed. If this quiet period results in a short nap, all the better. Limit the nap to twenty minutes to prevent sluggishness afterward.

P.S.:　The Irish poet and philosopher Joseph Campbell once said, "You must have a certain hour of the day or so where you do not know what was in the morning paper, a place where you simply experience and bring forth what you are, and what you might be."

The great philosopher, scientist, and moralist Blaise Pascal wrote in 1670: "All the troubles of men are caused by one single thing, which is their inability to stay quietly in a room."

32

Meditate

Common Opinion: *Meditating* means sitting uncomfortably upright on the floor with your legs strangely crossed as the odor of incense wafts about you.

Medical Opinion: Meditation is one of many ways to reduce stress.

Psychologist and spiritual teacher Joan Borysenko explains that meditation is simply intentional concentration on one thing. "Perhaps you have become so absorbed by gardening, reading, or even balancing your checkbook that your breathing slowed and you became as single-pointed as a panther stalking her dinner," she writes.

Yoga is another method of relaxation. Although I have no personal experience with yoga, many of my fellow physicians swear by it. They tell me there are both emotional and physical benefits. Having watched several videotapes demonstrating yoga, I can attest that it strengthens the muscles, stretches out tightened muscles, and most likely would put you at ease. Yoga classes are readily available at local health clubs and community centers. Also many good programs on videotape may be purchased or rented. You might even enjoy reading *Yoga Journal.*

Tai chi is a series of mind and body exercises that involves meditation, stretching, synchronized breathing, and shifting body weight. The movements are slow, controlled, and rhythmic. Advocates of tai chi report that it gives them a sense of peace and increased energy. It may also, Drs. Buckwater, Mooney, and Buckwater pointed out in the 1998 *Archives of The American Academy of Orthopedic Surgeons*, "improve balance and decrease the risk of falls" among the elderly.

Simple Change: Contemplate your navel. Give your undivided attention to a piece of chocolate cake. Analyze your putting stroke. Practice jazz scales. Whatever brings you satisfaction and serenity, just do it!

P.S.: For me, meditation is spending twenty to thirty minutes alone on a practice green concentrating on making twenty consecutive six-foot putts or practicing my trumpet in a private area in my basement. During these intervals of time, I block every other thought from my mind.

33

Work Crossword Puzzles, Play a Musical Instrument, or Play Cards

Common Opinion: Advancing age automatically brings marked decreases in mental function.

Medical Opinion: *Senile dementia* and *Alzheimer's disease* are degenerative diseases of the brain, just as arthritis is a degenerative disease of the joints and osteoporosis is a degenerative disease of the bones. Although there is inconsistent scientific validation, mental exercises may help prevent these degenerative disorders; there is strong evidence that the larger your memory bank, the longer it will take the degeneration of the neural pathways to occur.

It has been shown that different areas of the brain store different types of memory. Accordingly, various stimulation therapies may help memory.

Simple Change: Solving crossword puzzles is one stimulation therapy. You needn't try to work the Sunday *New York Times* puzzle to challenge your brain. Start with the puzzle in your daily newspaper. Have a dictionary and *Roget's Thesaurus* handy. Consult them regularly. Don't worry if you don't complete the puzzle. That's not important.

Another specific exercise for your brain is to learn to read music and play a musical instrument. If you played the piano or any instrument at a younger age, it might be easier to start with that instrument. On the other hand, maybe you've always wanted to learn to play a wind instrument or strum a guitar. There is a simple wind instrument that you can buy for about five dollars and learn to play a melody on the first day. It's called a recorder, or flutaphone. You can purchase one at most music shops.

Learning something new will promote a sense of self-worth and satisfaction. Card playing is yet another method of neurostimulation. Bridge, gin rummy, crazy eights, pinochle, spades, and euchre, are all possibilities. Play games that you enjoy. Play with your friends. Always volunteer to be the scorekeeper for the card game of your choice. It will make you a better player and at the same time sharpen your math skills.

P.S.:   Several years ago I started playing the trumpet again after a twenty-five-year hiatus. A few lessons, daily practice, and a week of adult band camp at Edinboro University in Pennsylvania soon brought me back to performing as I did at a younger age. More practice and more lessons have now enabled me to play in two local jazz bands. I also play in the summer with a community orchestra.

34

Play a Competitive Sport

Common Opinion: Playing a sport is just for exercise.

Medical Opinion: Recreation is one of the best methods of overcoming stress, even stress that you may not be aware of. Stress is lethal. Stress is a major factor in cardiovascular diseases, gastrointestinal disturbances, as well as emotional and mental disorders.

Simple Change: Choose the right activity that helps you relax. Each of us has different activities that help us overcome the stresses of everyday life. Pick one that truly does that. If you are frequently upset at the way you are hitting the golf ball, obviously golf is not the sport for you to reduce stress.

Then try to make that activity competitive. You might be surprised at the satisfaction it will give you. It may be a small bet, like a dollar for nine holes of golf, or just the satisfaction of scoring more points in a game of gin rummy. It will also make you concentrate more on the activity of the moment and allow you to forget the traumas of the day.

P.S.: For me, golf has always been the perfect release for the tension that has built up during a hectic week. It allows me to meet with friends I haven't seen for days, wear casual clothes, get outside in the fresh air, make that five-dollar Nassau bet, and get a little exercise. I get even more exercise if I don't use a golf cart.

35

Recognize Burnout and Deal with It

Common Opinion: *Burnout* is hard to define, even if you are experiencing it, and even harder to eliminate.

Medical Opinion: Burnout is when you wake up every morning as tired as you were when you went to bed. Burnout is when it's a real chore to prepare for work, face the traffic, engage in small talk with friends, or complete tasks that you do every day. Burnout is when you become agitated or enraged with only the smallest provocation. It's when you know there's something terribly wrong, but you can't for the life of you put your finger on it.

Burnout may reveal itself suddenly. Say you have been working on a large project. One morning you are unable to function as you've done every other day since the project began. Or burnout may be more insidious. It may gradually cause a decline in your energy, originality, ingenuity, and desire from years and years of living in the fast lane without taking time to "smell the roses."

To some degree, burnout has happened and will happen to you. The treatment, of course, is to alter your lifestyle, change your pattern, sidetrack, slow down, or "downshift," as business writer Amy Saltzman likes to say.

Simple Change: To overcome burnout, you first need to cultivate inner peace, well-being, happiness, and security. I recommend that you adhere to the six principles Sarah Ban Breathnach mentions in her book *Simple Abundance.*

These are the six threads of abundant living which, when woven together, produce a tapestry of contentment that wraps us in inner peace, well-being, happiness, and a sense of security. First, there is *gratitude.* When we do a mental and spiritual inventory of all that we have, we realize that we are very rich indeed. Gratitude gives way to *simplicity* – the desire to clear out, pare down, and realize the essentials of what we need to live truly well. Simplicity brings with it *order*, both internally and externally. A sense of order in our life brings us *harmony*. Harmony provides us with the inner peace we need to appreciate the beauty that surrounds us each day, and *beauty* opens us to *joy*.

36

If You Don't Like Something, Change It. If You Can't Change It, Change the Way You Think about It.

Common Opinion: If you have a bad temper or are easily frustrated, you just have to live with it.

Medical Opinion: Many mental problems, be it simple anger or frustration, or more serious problems like depression, are precipitated by habits. You *learn* to react to certain stimuli with specific patterns of mental activity. These patterns are the result of everything and everyone you have experienced since the day you were born. You can change either the stimuli (what you don't like) or your mental reaction to the stimuli (the way you think about it) by altering your habits. This is not easy. It takes practice. Yet it *can* be done.

In other words, you are the controller of your emotions. How many times have you said, "You make me mad"? What you are really saying is, "What you said or did was contrary to what *I* wanted you to say or do." Therefore, your reaction is to get mad. In this case, if you can't change the other person, then change your *reaction* to what he or she says or does. It's your responsibility to monitor your reactions, no one else's. The other person didn't make you mad. You made you mad.

People who live to be 100 years old share a common trait. They all knew about stress management before the term was coined. They tend not to fret or get upset. Most of them have a good sense of humor. In a recent New England study, it was found that centenarians tend to be low in neuroticism and high in conscientiousness. Even after suffering significant losses, they overcame emotional blows and forged ahead.

Simple Change: When you become frustrated by something in your environment, first think of a way to change what is disagreeable. If you conclude that there is no way to alter it so that it doesn't bother you, then change the way you *think* about it.

37

Be Monogamous

Common Opinion: Being monogamous is morally right but unrelated to good health.

Medical Opinion: Monogamy contributes significantly to good physical and mental health. Since your mate is your lifetime companion, he or she may be the strongest single factor in achieving a long, healthy life. You certainly need the encouragement and cooperation of your mate if you are going to alter certain habits and succeed with your new lifestyle. Since you will want your companion to be by your side for many years, you will probably want him or her to adopt the same lifestyle.

Having only one mate is a better method of disease prevention. Condoms are for contraception. They fail to prevent disease 15 percent of the time. In a recent medical journal, it was pointed out that the use of condoms may actually give a false sense of security in a high-risk situation. *HIV* is the number one cause of death among men ages 35 to 54. *AIDS* has been called the plague of the twenty-first century. This disease has the potential of wiping out the entire human population! The incidence of *syphilis*, *gonorrhea*, and *chancroid* (the three most common sexually transmitted diseases) has actually increased as medical technology has advanced in the United States. It would seem that the best prevention of sexually transmitted diseases would be for the medical community to promote strict monogamy. Even discounting diseases, evidence shows that one-on-one relationships contribute to longer and healthier lives.

Simple Change: To assure a harmonious relationship with your partner, vow today and every day to never take your mate's presence in your life for granted. Cultivate your love and friendship every day.

38

Think about Retirement Often

Common Opinion: You should delay making retirement plans until later in life, when you are closer to actually retiring.

Medical Opinion: Thinking sooner rather than later about retirement and all it has to offer can lessen the stress of your daily grind. Visions of freedom from time schedules alone may help to calm your frazzled nerves.

Simple Change: Decide what you will do with your time when you quit your present employment or profession. For some people, the best answer is to *not* retire at all. That's right, continue what you are now doing. Just change the amount of *time* you're doing it. Or, perhaps, change the *way* you are doing it. For example, you may prefer to act as an advisor or consultant in the line of work you are now doing. This will allow you to better manage your schedule.

If you choose to give up your type of work or profession completely, then plan ahead for what you will be doing day in and day out. Create a definite plan for each day. In my practice, I have seen a lot of people go directly into a sedentary lifestyle after leading very active pre-retirement lives. These people develop age-related illnesses and maladies much sooner than those who continue being active.

Start planning for your retirement early in your career so that you can enjoy your golden years free of financial worries. Even if you have followed all the advice for a long and healthy life, if you haven't planned for a financially sound retirement, you could lose the physical, mental, and emotional health you have obtained. Consult estate-planning experts *Now*.

A recent study by researchers at the University of Michigan, concludes that economic hardship affects people much like a major chronic disease. It will limit your physical and mental abilities. The longer the hardship, the more severe the impact on your health. Sustained economic hardship leaves physical, psychological, and emotional imprints that decrease the quality of daily life.

If your retirement plan includes a change of residence, make sure you are moving for the right reasons.

Don't think that changing your environment, in itself, will necessarily change your attitude. Jon Kakat-Zinn has written a book entitled *Wherever you go, there you are.* He points out that no matter where you go, the same mental habits will follow you. If you have a tendency to get upset and annoyed easily, or if you feel frustrated most of the time, or you're not satisfied with yourself, these tendencies will go wherever you go. On the other hand, if you are generally happy with yourself and your relationships with other people, then wherever you live you will show these same tendencies. Move to Florida if you want to. But remember, the people in Florida will probably affect you the same way as the people you now meet every day.

P.S.: A positive attitude toward your retirement years is very important for longevity. "I will never be an old man," said author, financier, and government advisor Bernard Baruch in 1955. "To me, old age is always fifteen years older than I am." He lived to the age of ninety-five.

My father was an avid deer hunter for eighty-eight years. He visited one particular mountain in northern Pennsylvania every year until his death. Hunting this mountain required a steep hike of one-and-a-half hours. Each ensuing year saw him taking longer and longer to reach the top, with more and longer rest periods. However, he knew that if he were able to "beat the hill" as he often repeated to me, he was going to live another year.

Retirement will be a big change. Think about it—often.

In Closing

Someone once offered me this good advice: "Be not the first by whom the new is tried, nor yet the last to lay the old aside."

Much of the advice in this book focuses on changing habits. This is essential if certain habits undermine your physical or mental health. Be careful, however, not to change your ways simply because doing so is fashionable. Remember another familiar saying: "If it's not broke, don't fix it."

Try new ideas, but never give up things that work for you.

About the Author

Joe Porter, a native of Ohio, is an orthopedic surgeon and team physician. He has practiced medicine for the past thirty years in central Ohio. Dr. Porter is a graduate of Muskingum College, where he obtained his bachelor of science degree; he is also a graduate of Ohio State University College of Medicine. For the past twelve years, Dr. Porter has participated in a medical assistance group, traveling frequently to Guyana, South America, to perform surgery for underprivileged citizens. In 1996, he received Rotary International's "Service Above Self" Award for his work in Guyana.

In his spare time, Dr. Porter is a musician and is active in community and regional theater as an actor and director. He and his wife, Tamara, have three children, two of whom are adults and one teenager. The Porters make their home in Zanesville, Ohio.

Please send:

_____ copies of _____
_____(*Title of book*)

at $ _____ each   TOTAL   _____

Nebr. residents add 5% sales tax   _____

Shipping/Handling
  $3.00 for first book.
  $1.00 for each additional book.   _____

        TOTAL ENCLOSED   _____

Name _____

Address _____

City _____ State ____ Zip _____

☐ Visa ☐ Master Card ☐ Am. Express

Credit card number _____

Expiration date _____

Order by credit card, personal check or money order.
Send to:

Addicus Books
Mail Order Dept.
P.O. Box 45327
Omaha, NE 68145
Or, order **TOLL FREE: 800-352-2873**

Please send:

_____ copies of _____
                                        (*Title of book*)

    at $ _____ each   TOTAL   _____

    Nebr. residents add 5% sales tax   _____

    Shipping/Handling
        $3.00 for first book.
        $1.00 for each additional book.   _____

            TOTAL ENCLOSED   _____

Name _____

Address _____

City _____ State ____ Zip _____

    ☐ Visa ☐ Master Card ☐ Am. Express

Credit card number _____

Expiration date _____

Order by credit card, personal check or money order.
Send to:

                        Addicus Books
                        Mail Order Dept.
                        P.O. Box 45327
                        Omaha, NE 68145
            Or, order **TOLL FREE: 800-352-2873**